H₂O Workouts®

Using the Pool Noodle

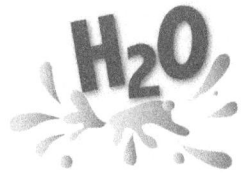

Francine Milford, LMT

Photographs by Paul and Francine Milford

ID: 978-1-105-83504-9

Caution
The techniques, ideas, and suggestions presented in this book
are not intended as a substitute for proper medical advice.
Any application of the techniques, ideas, and suggestions in
this book is at the reader's sole discretion and risk.

Please consult your health care provider before beginning this
or any other exercise program.

Cassiopeia Publishing

Fitness for the Next Generation

As more people are recognizing the need to live healthier and better lives, they have begun to set goals on how they will achieve and maintain a healthy body through proper nutrition and balanced work schedules.

Before long, the entire face of a typical aerobic class was changed as millions of people attempted to find a way to add exercise into their daily lives. Classes ranged in levels from easy senior workouts and classes for pregnant women to the high paced, high intensity Boot Camp classes.

Soon, many people were experiencing injuries from pushing their bodies too long and too far. When people are impatient to see results, they tend to exercise for long hours in a short period of time. Overuse injuries are one of the most common injuries found in the fitness industry.

Now most facilities offer Tai Chi, Qigong, Yoga and Pilates for people who want a good workout without the stress and strain of strenuous exercise.

The Great Equalizer

I call the water environment, the Great Equalizer. When I have taught water aerobic classes I would have ladies enter the water on crutches and even one came to class in a wheelchair. Once in the water, you could not tell the ladies apart. In the water environment, everyone is equal and everyone can receive a workout that is right for them and their fitness level.

In this book I will be sure to list exercises in **LEVELS**. If you are a beginner, then please stick to **Level One** exercises. As your body becomes familiar with the moves and becomes stronger, then move on up to **Level Two** and **Level Three**. Remember, don't overdue your workouts or you risk injuring your body and not being able to exercise at all. I would rather see you do a short ten minute workout everyday to build yourself up to the half hour or hour workout.

Be sure to get the approval of your primary health care physician before beginning this or any exercise routine.

Principles of Water Exercise

The water environment offers two important natural occurring effects to the water routine: buoyancy and resistance. Buoyancy is the property of being able to float. Buoyancy is also the power of a liquid to keep objects afloat; in this case, that object is you.

It is the natural ability of water to act as a cushion and in so doing, it protects you joints from injury, strain and re-injury. Many rehabilitation centers use the water environment in their treatment sessions.

While in the water environment, people can perform exercises they otherwise could not on land. Among these exercises are jumps, leaps, jumping jacks and pivots. Amazingly enough, the ability of water to be buoyant also allows water to provide resistance to water aerobics. Through changing direction, adding speed, or using longer levers, the water can provide a complete and thorough workout.

The water environment can become a natural total body workout. The more you put into your workout, the more you will receive from it. The faster you move, the harder the exercise becomes.

Water aerobics is also the perfect environment for those who are overweight or suffer from physical injuries. When you stand in water that is chest deep, you weigh only 10% of your normal body weight.

The water environment is also the great place to practice your golf or tennis swing. Even dancers and weight trainers can use the resistance in the water to build up muscles in a safe way.

Preparing to get Wet

When beginning your water exercise routine, the most important consideration is your swim suit. Find a suit that will cling comfortably to your body and still allow you freedom of movement.

Stay away from suits that will quickly fill with water with each jump that you take or that will ride up with each kick. If a suit isn't comfortable you will be fussing more with the suit than you will be concentrating on the exercises.

The second consideration is what to wear on your feet. Not everyone will be comfortable in wearing something on their feet while doing exercises in the water.

The bottom of the pool may be harsh on your feet through consistent movement. I haven't always had problems with this happening to my own feet, but it has happened, especially in backyard pools. You have plenty of choices to make when selecting what to wear on your feet. A pair of socks with good elastic is always an inexpensive purchase. I use a white booty sock that you will see later on in pictures in this book. I also own a pair of water socks (light shoes designed for walking in water) and a pair of water shoes. Yes, they actually look like tennis shoes but are made to go from land to water. I wear these shoes when I teach water aerobics as they add the perfect cushion for performing the moves on land.

There are also hand gloves, water buoys and pool noodles available to add resistance to your water workout. Many department stores and retail outlets now sell these products to water exercise enthusiasts. I highly suggest that you hold off on purchases until you have already begun your water workouts and find out whether or not you need more of resistance training, then make you purchase.

Tips for a Safe Workout

Do's and Dont's

- Do wear aqua shoes or aqua socks
- Do keep head in alignment of the spine.
- Do exercise in water that is of correct depth for you.
- Do relax and breathe slowly and deeply.
- Drink plenty of water before, during, and after exercising.
- Consult with your doctor before you begin exercising.
- Work at your own fitness level.
- Stop exercising if you feel faint, dizzy, nausea, or shortness of breath.
- Don't smoke or drink alcohol while exercising.
- Don't make fast, uncontrolled movements of the head or trunk in any direction.
- Don't use extreme range of motion.
- Don't use quick, jerky movement.
- Don't exercise with food or gum in your mouth.
- If you feel tired-stop
- For safety, there should be a lifeguard on duty during your workout or invite a friend to exercise with you.
- Never drink alcohol before, during, or immediately after a water workout.
- Perform your exercises in water that is chest high.
- Wait at least 1-3 hours after eating before working out
- When you enter the water that is cool, be sure to beginning walking, jogging, or bouncing right away to get your circulation moving.
- Always begin exercising slowly and then working up to more strenuous, energetic moves.
- Remember-Have fun!

Workout in Water

Warm-ups

As in any exercise program, it is important to prepare the body for the work that you are planning to put it through. We call this preparation, the Warm-Up.

In the Warm-Up you will increase the flow of blood to each and every muscle of the body. In this way, you will greatly reduce the risk of injury.

Warm-up exercises are usually gentle and slow activities that normally last 5 to 15 minutes. During this phase all the muscles and joints should be put through simple movements beginning with small range of motions and then increasing to larger, or full, range of motion.

In a typical land aerobic or workout class, we begin simply with marching in placing. The same holds true for water aerobics. In this chapter we will include several muscle groups that you will need to be sure you warm-up before beginning a water aerobics class. For some, this may be all the exercise that you can do in one day and if so, that is perfectly okay. What is important is move and stretch your body as often as you can throughout the day to keep it limber and lubricated.

When I received my certification in Aquatic Exercise, we practiced many types of water walking. Following a 3 to 5 minute warm-up exercise (such as marching in place) you could do some of the following walking exercises for the next 20-45 minutes:

- Walk forward and backwards
- Walk to the right and Walk to the left
- Walk in a big clockwise circle, then walk in a big counter-clockwise circle
- Walk on your toes
- Walk on your heels
- Walk like a crab sideways bouncing from flat feet with knees bent and open to the sides of your body.
- Walk forward and backward punching the water.

- Walk three steps and hop for one step.
- Do the Congo step in the water.
- Do the Bunny hop in the water.
- Do the Electric Slide in the water.
- Do your favorite Western Two Step in the water.
- Alternate between fast and slow walking to add intensity.
- Do the Soldier Walk, otherwise known on Goose Stepping
- Do Karate Kicks
- Walk doing knee lifts forward and front leg lift backwards
- Do Pendulum Swings with your legs side to side
- Do the Rocking Horse forward and backwards and change legs.
- Do Hamstring Curls forward and backwards.
- When stretching muscles in the warm-up phase it would be good if you could hold each stretch for at least 10 seconds (30 seconds is optimal).

Stretching
When performing the warm-up exercises and stretches, you should be able to feel slight warmth within your body. This is good and signals that you are preparing your body for the more vigorous workout that is to follow. The muscles that are stretched during the warm-up phase are the muscles that will be worked through the aerobic phase.

The Toe and Ankle Warm-ups
Some warm-up exercises and stretches can be performed inside, or at poolside, before you ever enter the water. If you find it difficult to spend more than 20 minutes in the water, then performing the warm-up stretches before entering the water may be a good idea.

The Toe and Ankle Warm-ups

Some warm-up exercises and stretches can be performed inside, or at poolside, before you ever enter the water. If you find it difficult to spend more than 20 minutes in the water, then performing the warm-up stretches before entering the water may be a good idea. Remember, do the best that you can but don't push your body beyond its physical limitation and most of all – Have Fun!

1. Toes and Ankles

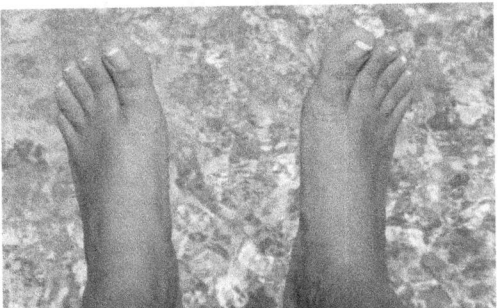

You can do this warm-up sitting in a chair before you enter the pool, or you may prefer to sit on the edge of the pool. Slowly point your toes towards you as far as you comfortably can, hold, and release. Do this exercise for a total of 8 repetitions. Fee the stretch from each toe as your attempt to bring each toe towards you and then release it.

2. Toes and Ankles

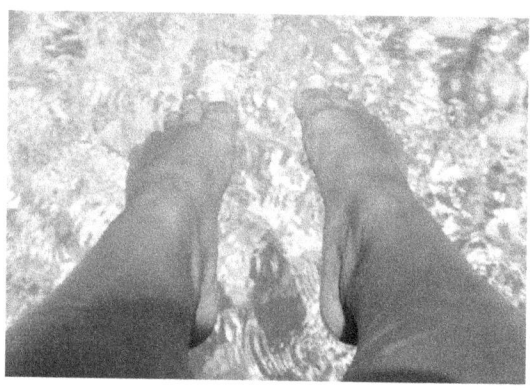

Press your toes away from your body, hold, and then relax the stretch. Perform this stretch for eight repetitions. Bring your focus to each of the toes and do not crunch them or fold them over one another. Allow each of the toes to enjoy and feel the stretch individually.

You will also be feeling a stretch in the front part of your leg, this is the anterior tibialis. When this muscle is not properly warmed up and stretched, many people suffer from Shin splints.

Do not over stretch this muscle.. The front of your leg should begin to feel warm.

3. Toes and Ankles

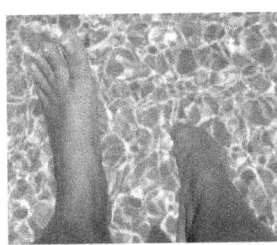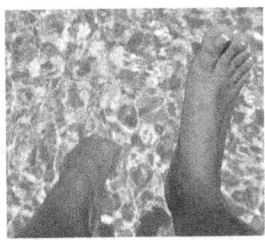

Alternate flexing and extending your feet. Press your right toes away from your body while you bring your left toes toward you body, hold for a few seconds, and then relax the stretch. Now, bring your right towed toward your body and press your left toes away from your body at the same time. Continue to alternate between your two feet in this way for a total of eight repetitions.

If you are sitting poolside, you can perform this exercise either outside of the water, or inside of the warm. The choice is up to you.

4. Toes and Ankles

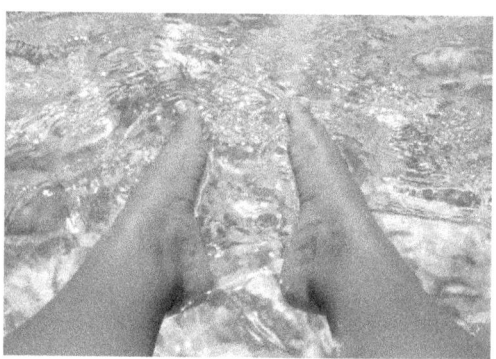

In the exercise above you will press the soles of your feet towards each other, hold for a few seconds, and then relax the stretch. Perform this stretch for eight repetitions.

Now, press the soles of your feet away from each other. Repeat for a total of eight repetitions. Bring your focus to each of the soles of your feet and do not crunch your toes or fold them over one another.

You will also be feeling a stretch in the front part of your leg, this is the anterior tibialis. When this muscle is not properly warmed up and stretched, many people suffer from Shin splints. The front of your leg should begin to feel warm, as well as, your ankles.

5. Toes and Ankles

Feet Swinging

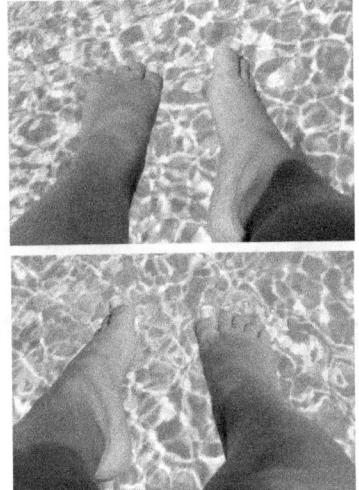

In the exercise above you will swing your feet to your right, hold for a few seconds, then swing your feet to the left, hold for a few seconds, and then relax. Perform these feet swinging exercises for eight repetitions.

Have fun with the exercise feeling the resistance of the water on your feet. Relax and enjoy.

6. Toes and Ankles

Circles

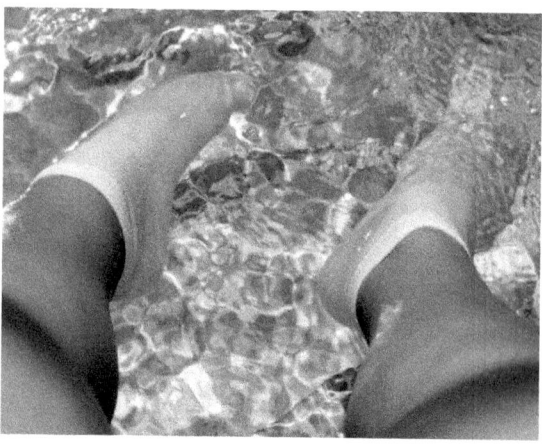

Using both feet at the same time, begin to move your feet in a circle clockwise. Begin by making eight small circles and then continue to enlarge each circle until you are making eight of the largest circles you can with you feet. Repeat the same exercise this time creating the smallest circles we can

Warm-ups for the Neck

Like the warm-ups for the toes and ankles, warm-ups for the neck can be performed on land before you enter the water environment. Do not push these stretches beyond what your physical capabilities are. Stretches should not be painful. If they are, stop immediately and consult with your primary health care provider.

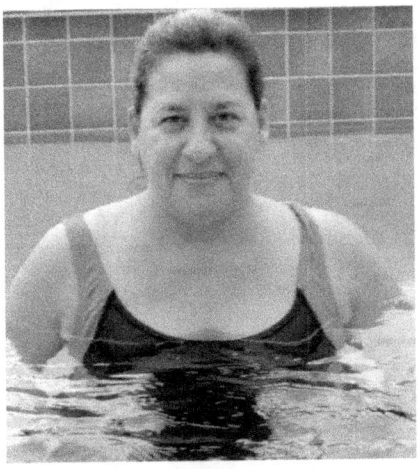

Starting Position

The starting point for the neck exercises will begin with the head in a neutral position as is shown in the diagram above, on the left. Keep you gaze in front of you at a slight angle downward. Be sure to breathe normally.

Neck Warm-ups

1. Neck

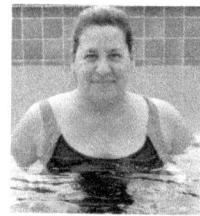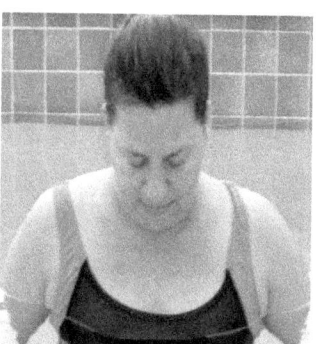

To Do:

With your head in the starting position take a nice deep slow breath in. As you exhale, slowly allow your head to fall forward touching your chin to your chest (note: if you cannot touch your chin to your chest, this is alright, don't force the movement.)

Now, slowly inhale and begin to return your head to the starting position. Repeat this exercise for a total of eight repetitions.

2. Neck

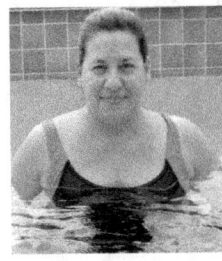
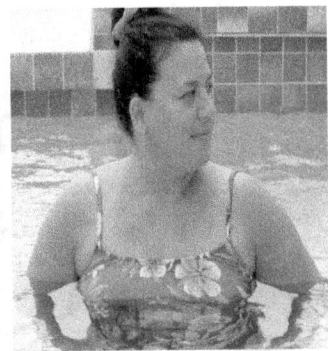

To Do:

With your head in the starting position take a nice deep slow breath in. As you exhale, slowly turn your head to left aligning your chin to over your left shoulder (note: if you cannot align your chin to over your shoulder, this is alright, don't force the movement.)

Now, slowly inhale and as you exhale, begin to return your head to the starting position.

With your head in the starting position take a nice deep slow breath in. As you exhale, slowly turn your head to right aligning your chin to over your right shoulder (note: if you cannot align your chin to over your shoulder, this is alright, don't force the movement.)

Repeat this exercise for a total of eight repetitions.

3. Neck

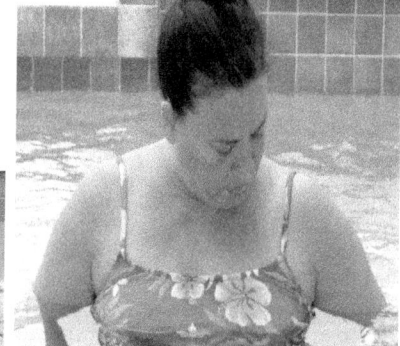
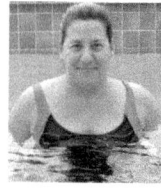

To Do:

With your head in the starting position take a nice deep slow breath in. As you exhale, slowly allow your chin to drop to the left to a point that is located half way between the center of your chest and your left shoulder (note: if you cannot touch your chin to your chest, this is alright, don't force the movement.) Now, slowly inhale and as you exhale, begin to return your head to the starting position.

With your head in the starting position take a nice deep slow breath in. As you exhale, slowly allow your chin to drop to the right to a point that is located half way between the center of your chest and your right shoulder (note: if you cannot touch your chin to your chest, this is alright, don't force the movement.)

Repeat this exercise for a total of eight repetitions.

4. Neck

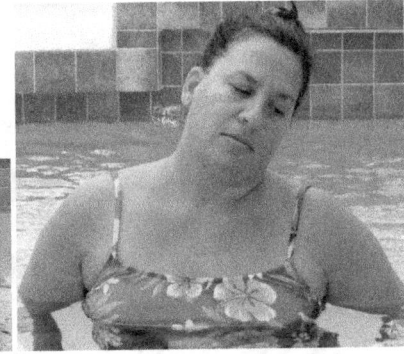

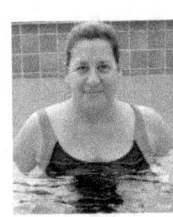

To Do:

With your head in the starting position take a nice deep slow breath in. As you exhale, slowly allow your left ear to drop to your left shoulder (note: if you cannot touch your ear to your shoulder, this is alright, don't force the movement.)

Now, slowly inhale and as you exhale, begin to return your head to the starting position.

With your head in the starting position take a nice deep slow breath in. As you exhale, slowly allow your right ear to drop to your right shoulder (note: if you cannot touch your ear to your shoulder, this is alright, don't force the movement.)

Repeat this exercise for a total of eight repetitions.

5. Neck

Head Rolls

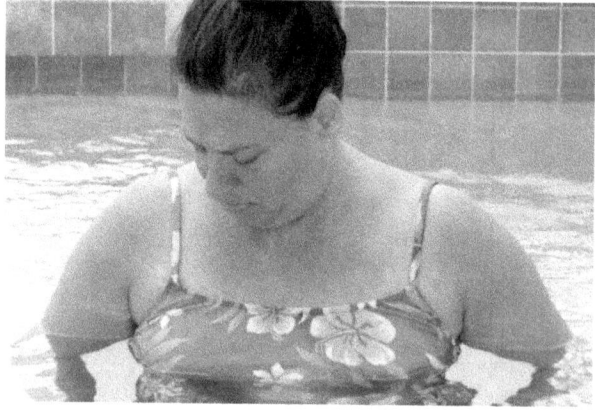

To Do:

Imagine that your nose is like the hands of wall clock. The numbers of the wall clock are right in front of your face. Take a nice deep slow breath in and as you slowly exhale you will begin with your nose in the twelve o'clock position. Moving clockwise outline the numbers of the clock from 3, to 6, to 9, and ending back at the top at the number 12 position. Repeat for eight repetitions.

Now, repeat the above exercise, this time moving counter clockwise beginning at the 12 position moving down to the 9, 6, 3, and back to the top 12 position. Repeat for eight repetitions.

Warm-up for the Shoulders

1. Shoulders

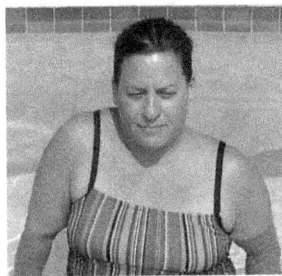 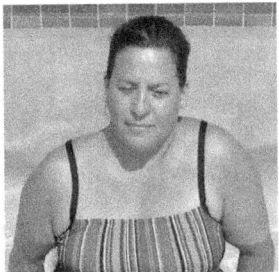

To Do:

Begin by planting both feet flat on the bottom of the pool. Bend your knees slightly and arms down at your sides. Now, standing perfectly straight, inhale and bring your right shoulder up to your right ear and hold. As you exhale release the shoulder back down to starting position. Remember-do NOT bring your ear down to meet the shoulder. This is very important. Repeat for a total of 8 repetitions. Now, inhale and bring your left shoulder up to your left ear and hold. As you exhale, relax and return to the starting position. Repeat for a total of 8 repetitions.

Alternating Shoulders: Inhale and bring your right shoulder up to your right ear and hold. Exhale and relax the shoulder back to the starting position. Inhale and bring your left shoulder up to your left ear and hold. Exhale and relax the shoulder back to the starting position. Repeat for a total of 16 repetitions.

2. Shoulders – Shrugs

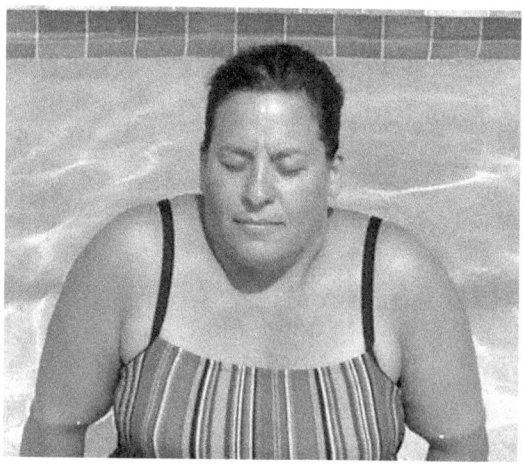

To Do:

Inhale and bring both of your shoulders up to your ears and hold for a few seconds. As you exhale, allow both shoulders to relax and return to the starting position. Continue for a total of 16 repetitions.

This is a great exercise to do throughout the day to reduce stress.

3. Shoulders – Circles

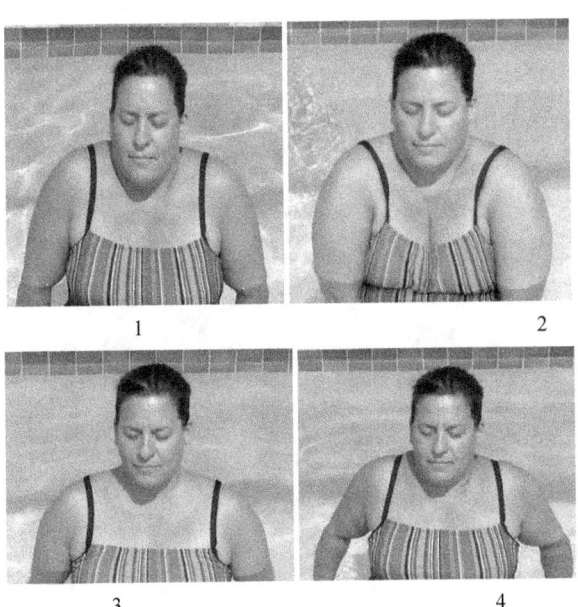

1

2

3

4

To Do:

Inhale and bring both shoulders up to your ears (1) and as you exhale allow the shoulders to push forward (2), then down (3), then back behind you (4) forming a circle. As you inhale again pull the shoulders back up to your ears and repeat the circle of exhaling and allowing the shoulders to drop to the front, down to the sides and to the back before returning up to the ears again. Repeat for a total of 8 repetitions.

When finished, repeat this exercise, this time inhaling and bringing the ears up to the shoulders and as you exhale, allowing the shoulders to drop towards the back, down to the sides, up to the front and back up to the ears in the next inhalation. (4-3-2-1). Repeat for a total of 8 repetitions.

5. Arms and Shoulders

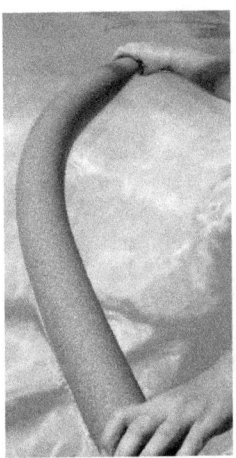 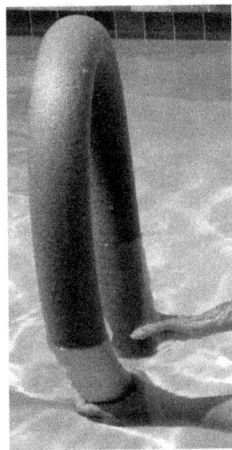

Starting Position

To Do:

Place your hands on the end of the pool noodle as far as is comfortable to you. Inhale, and as you exhale bring your hands, and the pool noodle, together in front of you. Hold and release to the starting position. Repeat for a total of eight repetitions. The slower you bring your hands together and apart, the harder the exercise.

6. Arms and Shoulders

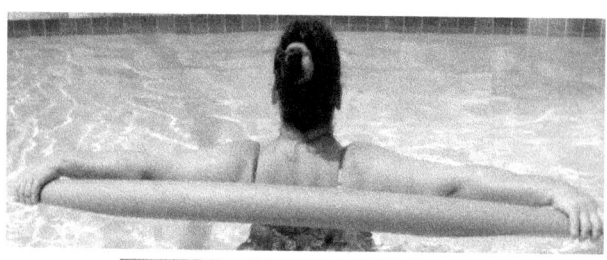

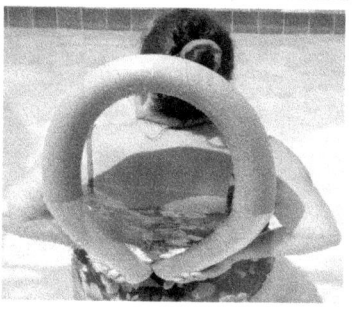

To Do:

Place your hands on the end of the pool noodle, behind your back, as far as is comfortable to you. Inhale, and as you exhale bring your hands, and the pool noodle, together in back of you. Hold and release to the starting position. Repeat for a total of eight repetitions. The slower you bring your hands together and apart, the harder the exercise. Do not strain your shoulders or cause pain.

7. Arms and Shoulders

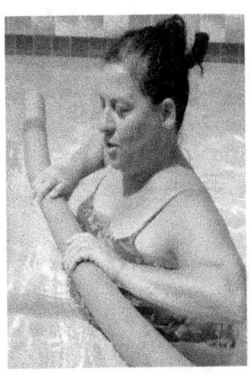 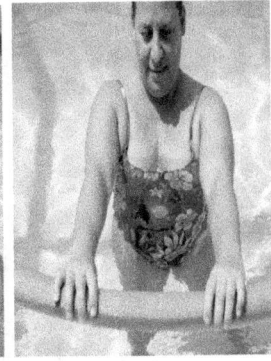

To Do:

Begin with feet firmly planted on the bottom of the pool and your knees slightly bent. Place both of your hands on the pool noodle in front of you at shoulder width apart.

Inhale, and as you exhale push the pool noodle away from your body as far as you can. Inhale and bring the pool noodle back to your chest. Continue to exhale and push the pool noodle away from you and inhale while bringing the pool noodle to your chest. Repeat for a total of at least eight repetitions.

8. Arms and Shoulders

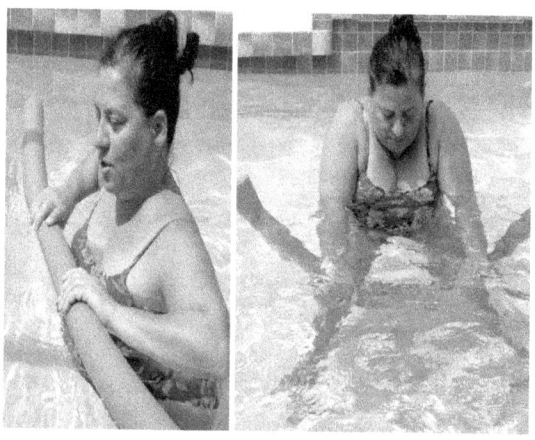

To Do:

Begin with feet firmly planted on the bottom of the pool and your knees slightly bent. Place both of your hands on the pool noodle in front of you at shoulder width apart.

Inhale, and as you exhale push the pool noodle down in front of your body as far as you can into the water. Inhale and bring the pool noodle back to your chest. Continue to exhale and push the pool noodle down into the water and inhale while bringing the pool noodle to your chest. Repeat for a total of at least eight repetitions.

9. Arms and Shoulders

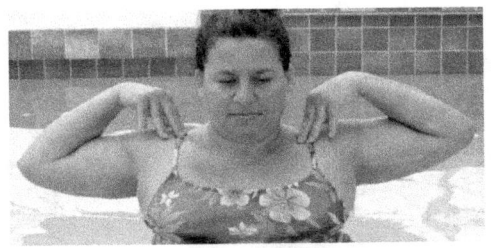

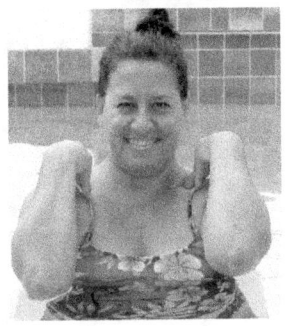

To Do:

Place your hands on your shoulder with elbows pointed outwards from your body as shown in the picture above. Now, slowly bring elbows towards the front of you body, hold, and release back to starting point. Do a total of eight repetitions.

10. Arms and Shoulders

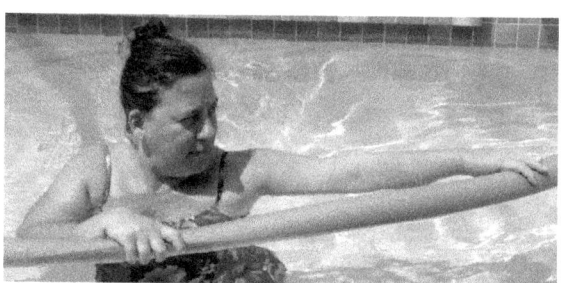

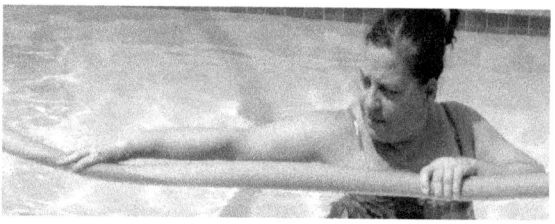

To Do:

Place both of your hands about 6-8 inches from the ends of the pool noodle where ever it is still comfortable for you without straining. Keep both feet on the bottom of the pool with your knees slightly bent. Inhale, and as you exhale, twist your body to the left as far as is comfortable. Inhale again and you exhale return to the starting position. Inhale and as you exhale, twist your body to the right as far as is comfortable. Inhale once more and as your exhale return to the starting position. Repeat for a total of eight repetitions.

11. Arms and Shoulders

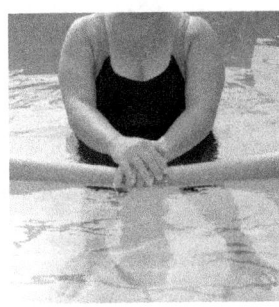 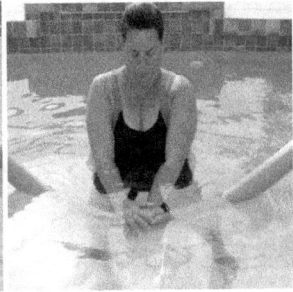

To Do:

Stand with feet on the bottom of the pool and with knees slightly bent. Place both hands (one over the other) at the center of the pool noodle.

Take a deep breath and as you exhale, press the hands (and pool noodle) down into the water as low as you can. Hold and release back to the starting position shown in the picture on the left top of the page.

To make this exercise as efficient as possible, lower and raise the pool noodle in the water as slow as you can. Repeat for a total of eight repetitions.

Note: If you feel any pain in your shoulders with this exercise, stop immediately.

12. Arms and Shoulders

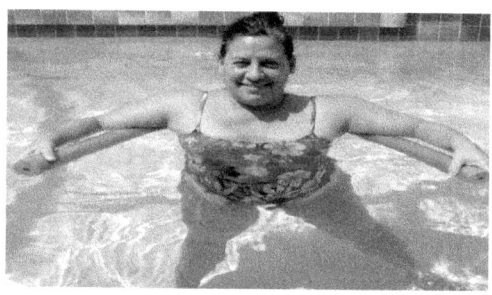

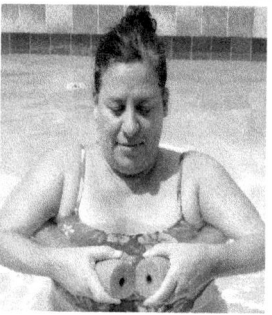

To Do:

Place the pool noodle behind your back and lay your arms over both ends of the noodle. Inhale and as you exhale bring both ends of the pool noodle together in front of you, hold for a few seconds, and slowly release back to the starting position. Repeat for a total of at least eight repetitions.

13. Arms and Shoulders

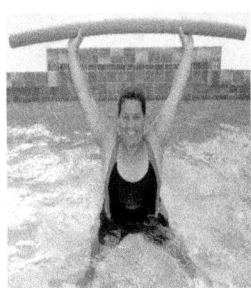 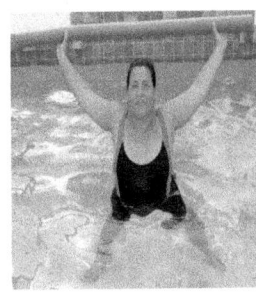

To Do:

Begin this exercise by standing with your legs more than shoulder width apart. Keep your feet planted firmly on the bottom of the pool with knees in a relaxed position.

Extend both of your arms straight over your head in front of your ears. Inhale. As you exhale, slowly bring your arms, holding on to the pool noodle, backwards. Keep your upright position and just allow your arms to fall back as far as they can go without over stressing them. Hold the position for a few seconds and release back to the starting position. Repeat for a total of eight repetitions.

This stretch will add a nice stretch in through the muscles of the chest and abdominal area.

Warm-up for the Wrists

Note: If you have any wrist problems or injuries-please consult your health care provider before beginning these exercises.

Wrist Starting Position

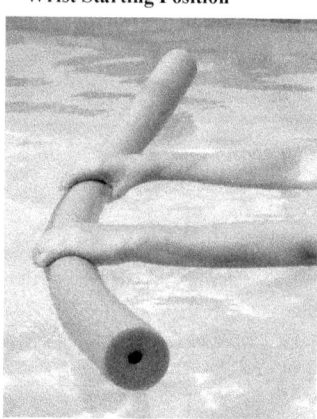

Starting Position:

   Begin the following exercises in the starting position as shown in the picture above on the left. To begin, make sure that both of your feet are planted firmly on the bottom of the pool with knees slightly bent. Be sure that your knees are shoulder width apart.

   Extend both of your arms straight out in front of your body with fingers pointing away from your body. Keep your arms straight but do not lock your elbows. Keep a soft, but firm grip on the pool noodle. This is the starting position.

1. Wrist

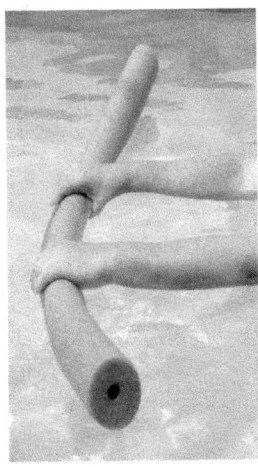 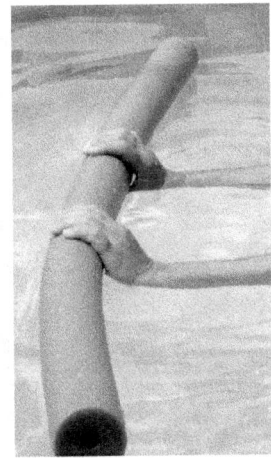

To Do:

Take a nice slow, deep breath and at the same time, lift the fingers of both of your hands towards you while keeping the heel of your hand pushing away from your body, hold the stretch for a few seconds.

As you slowly exhale, lower your fingers back to the starting position as shown in the picture above, on the left.

Repeat for a total of eight repetitions.

2. Wrists

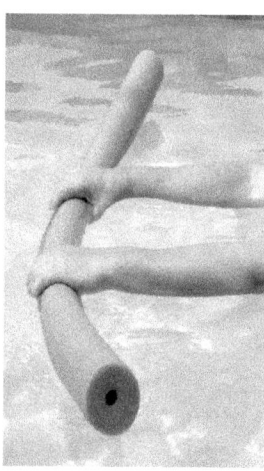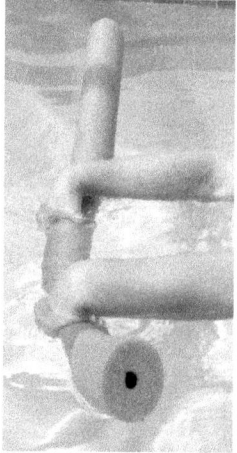

To Do:

Extend both of your arms straight out in front of your body. Do not lock your elbows. If this is uncomfortable, just relax your arms and do the best that you can. Take a nice slow, deep breath and at the same time, point the fingers of both of your hands down towards the bottom of the pool, while keeping your arms extended away from your body, hold the stretch for a few seconds.

As you slowly exhale, raise your fingers back to the starting position as shown in the picture above, on the left. Repeat for a total of eight repetitions.

Finger Exercises

Starting Position

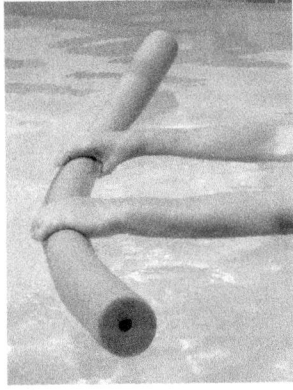

To Do:

To perform the following finger exercises you will need to begin in the starting position as shown below. You will place you hands on the pool noodle at about shoulder width apart. Keep your knees bent and breathe regularly. Start with the index finger of both of your hands and apply slight pressure to the pool noodle, hold and count to eight, then release the pressure. Continue to press, hold and count, and release for a total of eight repetitions.

Repeat the entire process using your middle finger, the ring finger and ending with the little pinkie finger. If you feel uncomfortable or experience any pain, stop immediately.

Index Finger   **Middle Finger**

Ring Finger   **Pinkie**

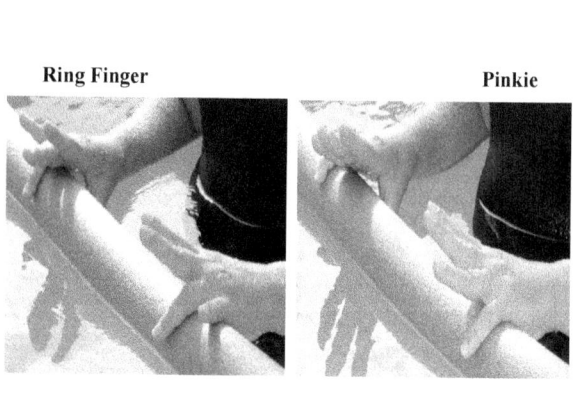

Basic Water Moves

1. Knee-ups

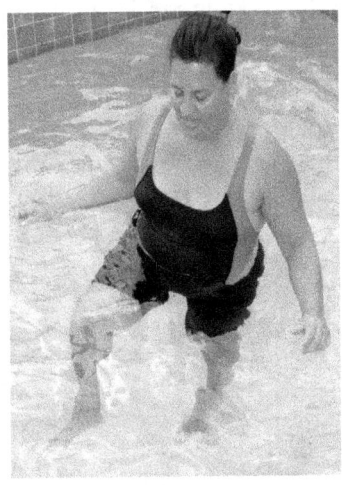

Knee-ups

Begin with both of your feet firmly planted on the bottom of the
pool. Now, as you are balancing yourself, lift your right knee up as
high as you can. Do not go over a 90 degree angle. Press your right
foot back to the bottom of the pool and straighten out your leg. Do
this for a total of 8 repetitions and repeat the whole exercise on your
left leg. Work at a nice, steady, and slow speed. Take your time.
Work up to 25 repetitions on each leg.

Knee-ups - Level One

Walk slowly forward and backward from one side of the pool to the other side. The faster you walk, the more intense the workout will be. Try to keep the pace slow and steady so that you can keep your balance without too much stress on your body.

Knee-ups - Level Two

Increase the rate of speed that you are using to lift and lower each knee. The faster you can safely lift and lower your knee, the harder the workout will be. You can call it 'Power Walking' if you like. Move your arms through the water at your side as you try to walk briskly forward and backward. Don't overdo this exercise as you will quickly discover that it will tire you out and increase your heart rate very rapidly.

Knee-ups - Level Three

1. **Alternate Knee Lifts-**For this exercise you will alternate between lifting the right knee and lifting the left knee. The exercise will be "Right knee up, right knee down, Left knee up, left knee down." Repeat this for a total of 16 repetitions. Alternate the rate of speed that you are using to perform this

2. **Running in Place-**Should you be able to alternate the speed of your leg lifts enough, you will be able to start running in place. Do this for 30 seconds working up to a minute or more. To add variety and intensity, practice running at different rates of speed for a great workout.

3. **Running with Movement-**Add direction. Run forward as far as you can, then run backward as far as you can. Do this for 8 repetitions. Run in a clockwise circle, then switch direction and run in a counterclockwise circle. Do this for several repetitions on each side.

2. Alternating Knee Lifts

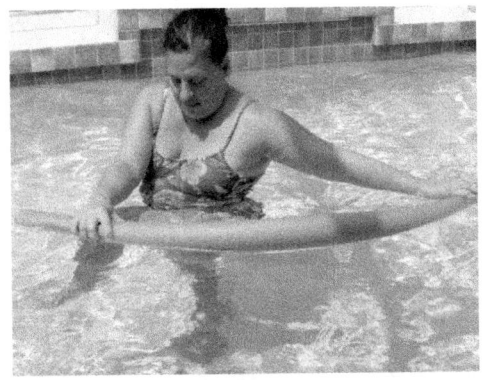

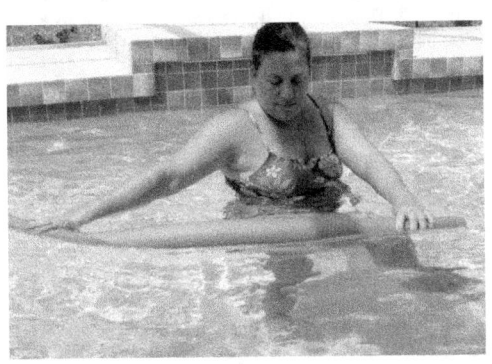

Single Knee Lifts- Level One

Begin with both of your feet firmly planted on the bottom of the pool. Lift your right knee up toward the left side of your body and bring your pool noodle over to touch the right knee. Return the right foot back down to the bottom of the pool and straighten up your body.

Repeat bringing the right knee up and towards the left side of the front of your body for a total of 8 repetitions, and then repeat the entire exercise using the left knee and the right side of your body.

Be sure to make your movements slow and deliberate. Do not throw your body out of alignment or contort your body needlessly. Inhale as you straighten and exhale as you bring the elbow to the knee. Work up to 25 repetitions on each knee.

Alternating Knee Lifts - Level Two

In Level Two you will do the same exercise as listed in Level One but you will alternate the right and left knees. The exercise will go like this: "Left knee up towards right side of body, right knee up towards left side of body, and straighten up. You will do this for a total of 16 repetitions. Work up to 25 repetitions.

Alternating Knee Lifts - Level Three

You will now do the alternate knee lifts as described in Level Two but at a faster rate of speed. You will feel like you are running and you feet may not come fully down on the bottom of the pool. To add variety and intensity, alternate between slow and fast rates of speed, this will help to build up your heart rate. If you like, you can move forward and backward while doing this exercise.

3. Front Leg Lifts

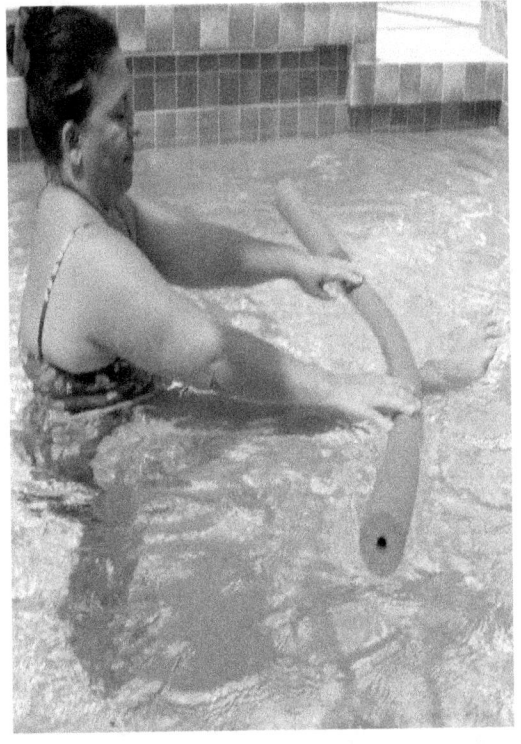

Front Leg Lifts – Level One

Begin with both feet planted firmly on the bottom of the pool and with your knees soft. Now, inhale and bring your left leg straight up in front of you as high as you comfortably can, hold for a few seconds, and then as exhale, bring your leg back down to the starting position. Repeat for a total of eight repetitions.

When finished, repeat the entire exercise with your right leg for a total of eight repetitions.

Front Leg Lifts - Level Two

Begin in the starting position listed above. This time you will alternate lifting your left leg and returning it to the starting position and then lifting your right leg and returning it to the starting position. Continue alternative the front leg lifts for a total of 16 repetitions.

Front Leg Lifts – Level Three

Repeat this exercise as listed in Level Two only add speed, hopping from right to left leg. You can also move forward and backward while alternating front leg lifts.

4. Side Leg Lifts

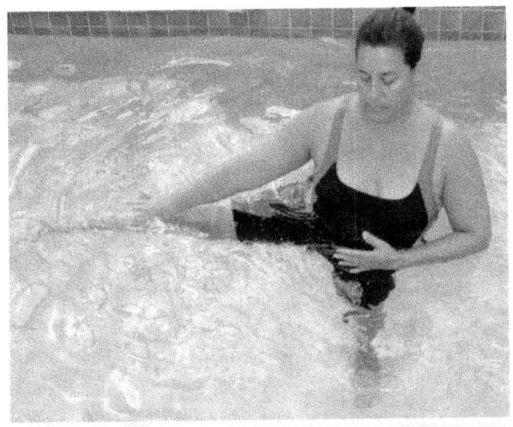

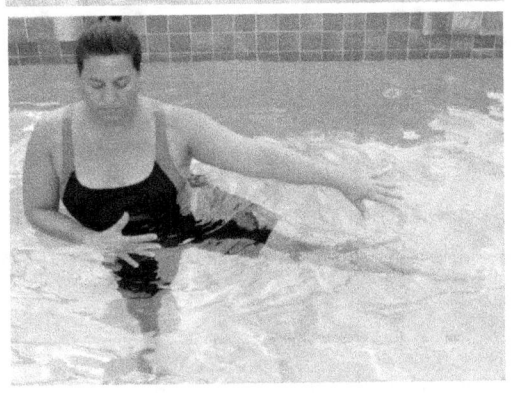

Side Leg Lifts – Level One

Plant both of your feet firmly on the bottom of the pool and keep your knees soft. Now, inhale and lift your right straight up at your side as high as you comfortably can, hold for a few seconds, and then exhale and release the leg back to the starting position. Repeat for a total of eight repetitions. When finished, repeat the entire exercise on your left leg for a total of eight repetitions.

Side Leg Lifts - Level Two

Plant both of your feet firmly on the bottom of the pool and keep your knees soft. Now, lift your right leg up as far as you can to your right side and return to the starting position. Then, lift your left leg up as far as you can to your left side and return to the starting position. Repeat alternating between the right leg and the left leg for a total of 16 repetitions.

Side Leg Lifts – Level Three

Add speed to the exercise shifting rapidly between the right and left leg lifts. You can also move forward and backward as you do this exercise. As an added treat, do this exercise while moving sideways from one end of the pool to the other. You can vary your speed and even add a double hop on one foot to add variety to your workout.

Play some upbeat music while you are exercising and 'dance' to the music while you are doing your water workout. Match your speed and movements to the songs you have chosen to alleviate any boredom you may suffer from exercise.

With music, you see the time fly by very quickly. Be sure to pick music that makes you want to move and if you can sing along with the words, all the better.

5. Touch Foot in Front

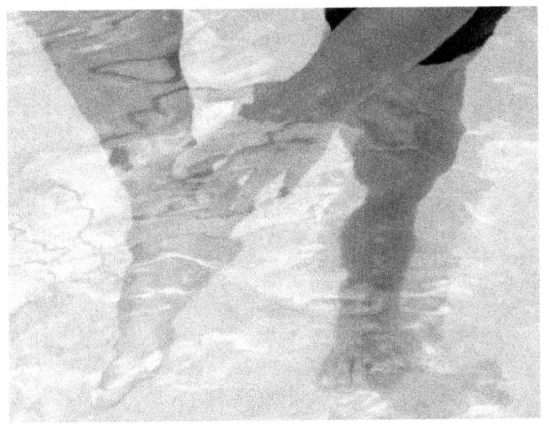

Touch Foot in Front - Level One

For this exercise you will bring your right foot up in front of your body and you will reach down into the water with your left hand to touch the right foot. Straighten up and repeat again bringing your right foot up to the front of your body and touching it with your left hand. Repeat this exercise for at least 8 repetitions, building to 25.

When finished, repeat this exercising bringing your left up in front of your body and reaching down with your right hand to touch your foot. Straighten up and repeat the exercise again for a total of 8 repetitions, building to 25. Keep a nice, slow and steady pace. If you can't touch your foot, that is alright. Just do the best that you can.

Touch Foot in Front - Level Two

      To add intensity to movement described in level two we will alternated the feet. The directions will be as follows: "Right foot up, left hand down, Left foot up, right hand down."

Touch Foot in Front - Level Two

      You can also increase the intensity of this movement by adding speed creating a hopping effect from foot to foot. The faster you go, the higher the intensity. Repeat for 16 to 25 repetitions.

      Repeat this entire exercise by touching your hand to your feet behind you. This is very difficult to do and you may find that you cannot touch your foot to your opposite hand at all. This is okay. Just do the best you can do without straining or injuring yourself.

Touch Foot on Pool Noodle (Alternate Movement)

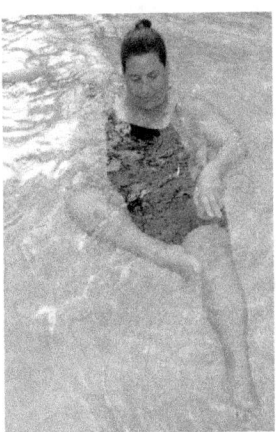 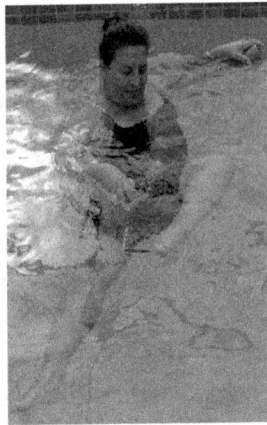

Touch Foot in Front - Level One

Perform this exercise while laying back on your pool noodle and bend your right knee and bring your right foot up to the front of your body and touch it with your right hand while holding on to the pool noodle. Try to touch your foot, then straighten up your body, and repeat the exercise again on the same foot for 8 repetitions. Build up to 25 repetitions.

When finished, repeat the entire exercise using your left foot and your right hand. Do not strain or twist your back in order to do these exercises. Do what is comfortable for you.

Please note that you do not have to actually touch your foot in order to derive some benefits from this exercise. Just do the best that you can do.

Touch Foot in Back - Level Two

To build intensity in this movement you can begin by alternating the left foot and right hand and right foot and left hand. The directions will be: "Left foot up, right hand down, Right foot up, left hand down." Repeat for 16 to 25 repetitions.

Touch Foot in Back - Level Three

To increase the intensity of this exercise even more, add speed to the movements. You will feel like you are hopping from one foot to the other. You can also add varying speeds to this exercise to make it feel more intense.

7. Inner/Outer Thigh Work

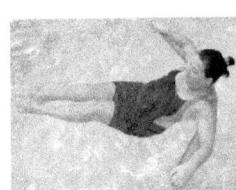 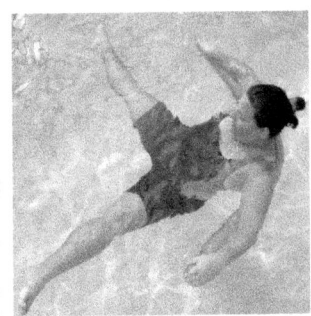

Level One

Begin by leaning back comfortably on your pool noodle and allowing your feet to float up in front of you as shown in the picture above on the left. Inhale and spread your legs as far apart as you comfortably can as shown in the above picture on the right. Exhale and bring your legs back together again. Do eight times.

Level Two

When finished, turn around in the pool and face the opposite direction. Repeat the above exercises as listed in the exercise above.

NOTE: This exercise in Level two could be very hard and put undue stress on your back. If you suffer from back injuries and problems, please do not perform this exercise.

8. Knees In

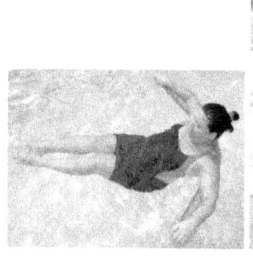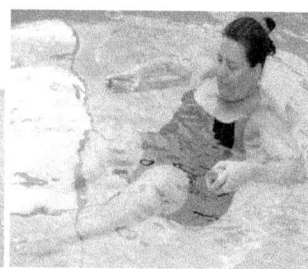

Knees in – Level One

Begin by leaning back comfortably on your pool noodle and allowing your feet to float up in front of you as shown in the picture above on the left.

Inhale and bring both knees towards your chest. As you exhale, push both feet away from your body. Continue bringing knees in towards your chest and pushing them away for at least eight repetitions. Be sure to press the heels of your feet away from your body.

Knees in - Level Two

For level two, you will perform the exercise as listed in level one only you will add speed to the movement. The faster you switch your legs, the harder and more intense the exercise will become.

You can also add variety to the movement by fast and slower movements together.

9. Abdominal Twists

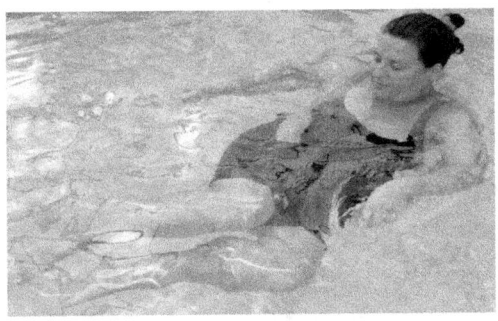

Abdominal Twists – Level One

Begin by leaning back comfortably on your pool noodle and allowing your feet to float up in front of you as shown in the picture above on the left.

Inhale and bring both knees to your chest and as you exhale, twist your body, along with your knees to the right. Inhale and twist your body back to the center and as you exhale, extend your legs away from your body as in the starting position in the top picture. Repeat for a total of eight repetitions on the right side of your body and then perform the entire exercise on the left side of your body.

Abdominal Twists - Level Two

Repeat the same exercise as described above only add speed to the twists. The faster you bring your knees in to your chest and back out, the more intense the workout will be.

10. Bicycles

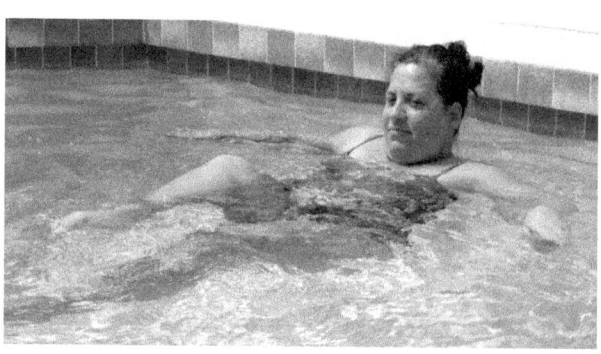

Level One

Lean back on your pool noodle and alternate bringing each knee to your chest and then pushing it away, imitating the movement of pedaling a bicycle. Continue pedaling for at least 16 repetitions,.

Level Two

Repeat the exercise above but add speed and movement to increase the intensity of this exercise. You can also alternate between pedaling forward and pedaling backward.

Level Two

Increase intensity by adding ankle weights or buoys to your ankles.

Bicycle Alternative Exercise

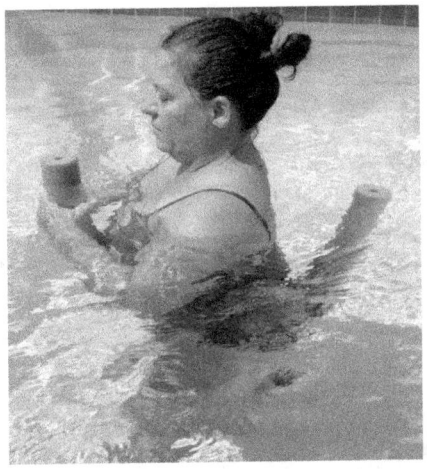

To Do:

Straddle your pool noodle making sure that the pool noodle is equal in length on both the front and back sides of your body. Pretend that you are sitting on a bicycle and begin to pedal bringing alternate knees to your chest. Pedal forward and backward.

Level Two

You can add intensity to this movement by adjusting your rate of speed and the size of the circles in your pedaling.

11. Frog

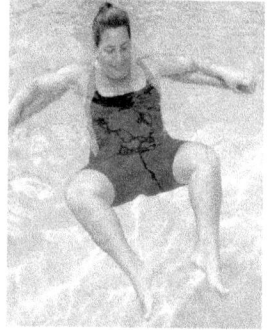

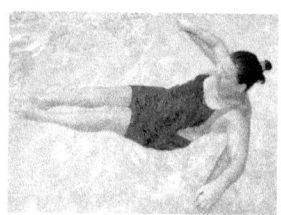

To Do:

Begin this exercise as shown in the photograph on the top left of the page by relaxing back on the pool noodle and allowing both your feet and legs to float up to the top of the water.

Inhale, bend your knees, and bring the heels of both of your feet towards your body. As you exhale, extend both of your legs back to the starting position, pointing your toes.

Repeat inhaling and bringing the heels of your feet towards your body, and exhaling and extending your legs back out in front of you. Continue for at least eight repetitions.

Stretches

1. Shoulder Stretch

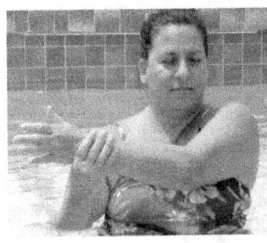 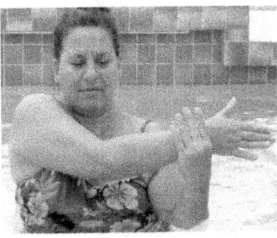

1   2

To Do:

Begin the cool down by bring your straight left arm across the front of your body and gently grasp your left wrist with your right hand (as shown in picture #1). Gently press the left arm toward your right arm.

Be sure to keep your hips and body straight and looking forward. Do not force the stretch and be sure to inhale and exhale freely and easily. Release the arm.

Now, take your straight right arm and bring it across the front of your body and gently grasp your right wrist with your left hand and press the arms towards your left arm (as shown in picture #2). Release the arm. Repeat on both sides for an additional two more times.

2. Shoulder Hug

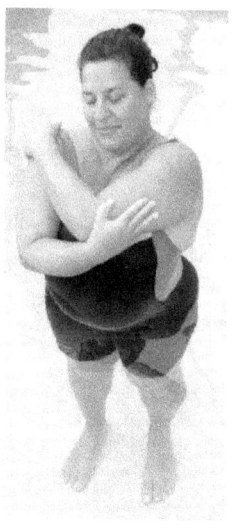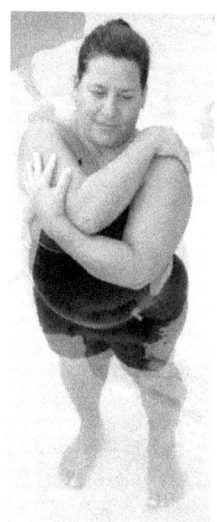

To Do:

A great shoulder stretch in the 'hug'. Just wrap your arms around each other and give yourself a big hug. Inhale and exhale freely and easily.

Release your hug and switch your arms around and give yourself another big hug. Inhale and exhale freely and easily. Repeat the hug for an additional two more times on each side.

3. Tricep Stretch

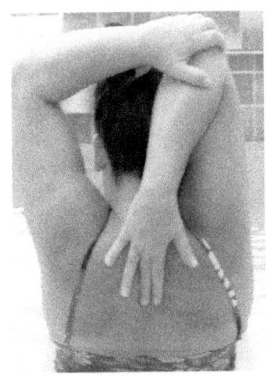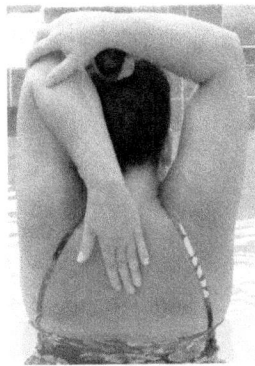

To Do:

Bring your right arm straight out in front of your body and reach upward. Bend the elbow and bring the right hand down to lay flat on your back with the palm of your right hand on your back.

Bring your left hand over and place it on your right elbow. Gently add pressure to your right elbow to push it backward giving you a stretch in your triceps muscle. Breathe normally.

Release your arm and bring your left arm straight out in front of your body and reach upward. Bend the elbow and bring the left hand down to lay palms flat on your back.

Bring your right hand over and place it on your left elbow. Gently add pressure to your left elbow and push it backward giving you a stretch in your triceps muscle. Breathe normally. Continue stretching the triceps for an additional two more times.

4. Lat Stretch

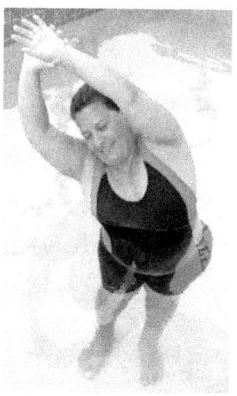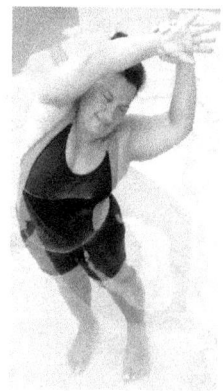

To Do:

Begin this exercise by standing with feet flat on the bottom of the pool and shoulder width apart. Reach your left arm straight upward from your body. Inhale and clasp your left wrist with your right hand. As you exhale, gently pull the left hand, and arm, down towards the right. Inhale and return to starting position and exhale and release.

Inhale again. This time extend your right arm straight upward from your body. Inhale and clasp your right wrist with your left hand. As you exhale, gently pull the right hand, and arm, down towards the left. Inhale and return to starting position and exhale and release. Repeat this exercise for a total of at least 8 stretches.

5. Hip Stretch

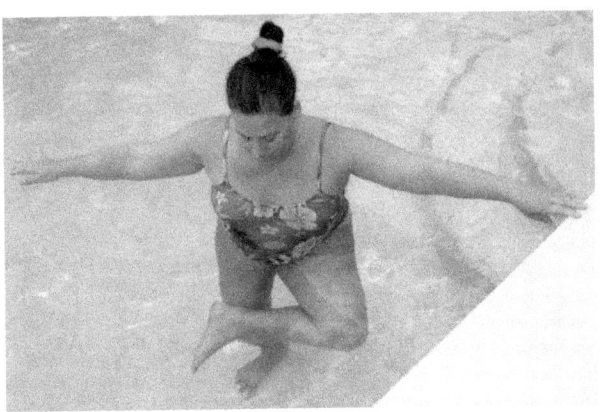

To Do:

Stand with both of your feet planted firmly on the bottom of the pool shoulder width apart. Bend your left knee and bring your left up the front of your body and place it just above your knee.

Now, as you exhale, slowly bend your right knee and allow yourself to sink into the water as far as you can comfortably go. Hold, and then release into starting position. Repeat this exercise on the other side using your right foot on your left thigh.

To add more depth to this hip stretch exercise you can do the following: As you sink into the water as far down as you can go, hold that position and lift up off the heel of your foot.

6. Side Stretch

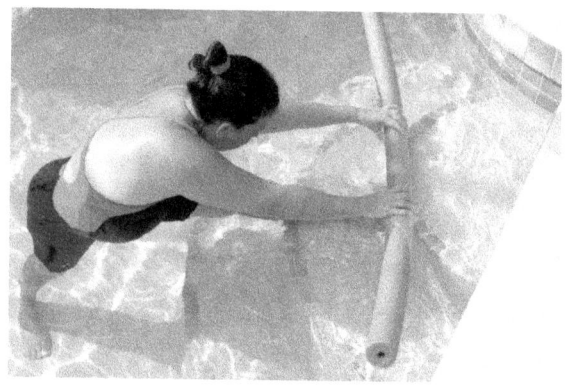

To Do:

Begin by standing in front of a pair of stairs in the pool, or on any graded surface. Lift one leg up to wherever is comfortable to you and to your fitness level. Inhale. As you exhale, slowly slide the pool noodle down to the top of your foot (or as close to your feet) as you can.

Inhale and bring your body back up to a straightened position. Repeat the exhalation and stretch forward and the inhalation, straightening back to starting position. Repeat for a total of eight repetitions and then place your opposite leg on the step and repeat the stretch for an additional eight repetitions.

7. Body Stretch

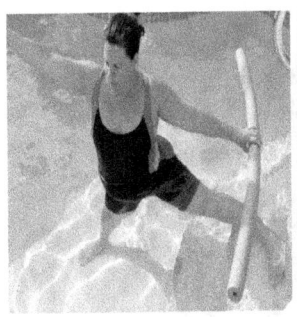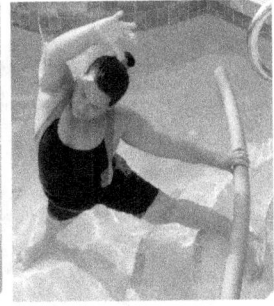

To Do:

Start with your feet planted firmly on the bottom of the pool sideways to a step or slope in the pool (you can always use a pool bench if you like). Lift the left foot, which is closest to the step, up and place it sideways on the step as shown in the picture above left.

Now, inhale and lift your right arm straight into the air. As you exhale, bring the right arm down over your right ear towards the left foot. Be sure to bend at the waist to reach as far as is comfortable to your fitness level.

Do not strain through this exercise. Inhale back up to starting position and exhale back down towards the foot. Continue for at least eight repetitions. When finished, turn around and place your right foot on the step and lift your left arm into the arm and repeat the above exercise for an additional eight repetitions.

Balance-Finding your Core

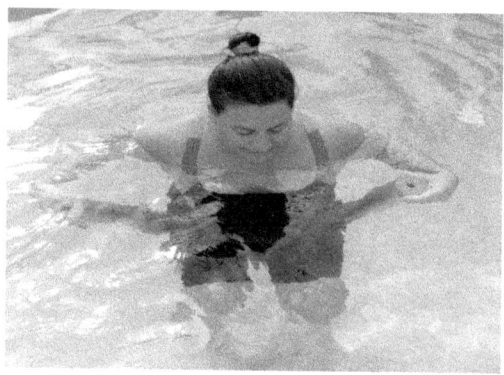

To Do:

      This is a great exercise movement to help strengthen the core of your body while improving your balance and focus. Sit on the center of your pool noodle allowing each end to be equal in length. Now relax and allow your body to find a peaceful rhythm where you can stay afloat and upright. This is a great exercise for the abdominal muscles that will work to keep you steady against the natural currents of the pool or water.

      Find a focal point and allow your mind to sit in that focal point. Inhale and exhale smoothly, slowly and deeply. Try to clear your mind of all outside annoyances and distractions. Enjoy the moment.

Cool Down

Cool Downs are a series of movements that are used after an exercise class as a means to return the heart rate back to its normal pre-exercise rate. The more you exercise, the stronger your heart and lungs will become and the shorter the period of time it will take for the heart rate to return to normal. If you need help in adapting any of these exercises to your own specific limitations, just drop me an email at RevReikiND@cs.com and we can discuss options.

Cool Down

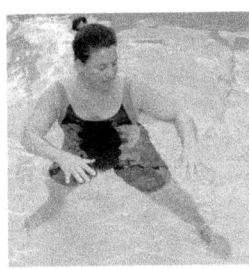 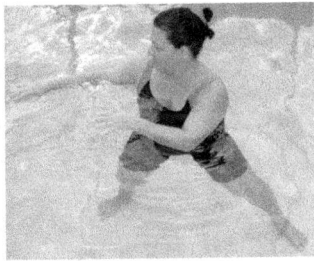

To Do:

You can add mindfulness and Breathwork to this cool down exercise. To do this exercise, spread your legs apart as far as you comfortably can to maintain your body's balance in the water.

Place your hands, palm down, at the very top of the water and pretend that there are flower petals floating on the top of the water. Gently push the flower petals to the left and then to right trying not to disturb the petals, or the water.

About the Author

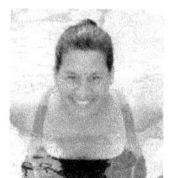

Francine Milford has had a very long career in the Fitness Industry. Working for more than twenty years in a variety of sports and exercise related classes, she is also an avid walker and enjoys reading a book audio tape while bicycling around the neighborhood.

A national and state licensed massage therapist and personal trainer, Francine has achieved certifications through the YMCA S.A.F.E. Aerobic Program, AEA Aquatics Exercise Association, ESA Exercise Safety Association, and AFAA Aerobics Fitness Association.

Francine has also received the Tai Chi for Arthritis Certification having studied under Dr. Paul Lam, as well as, 180 hours of professional training in Tai Kwan Do. She has taught such classes as Kick Boxing, Bench Stepping, Low Impact Aerobics, High Impact Aerobics, Basic Floor and Senior Aerobics and all types of Water Aerobic classes.

As a fitness specialist, Francine has been hired to lead classes and workshops at offices, condo organizations, clubs and private groups.

Having spent the last ten years working with the senior population, Francine has developed exercises that are both safe and effective for those with physical limitations. Visit online at www.H2OWorkouts.com.